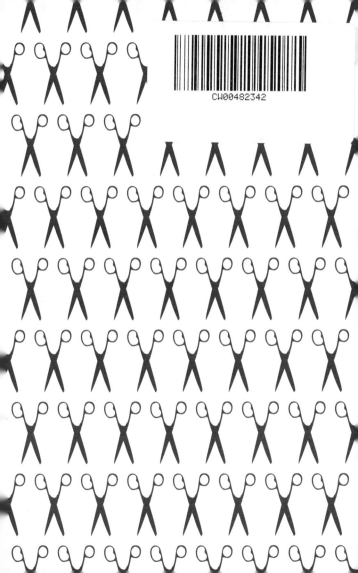

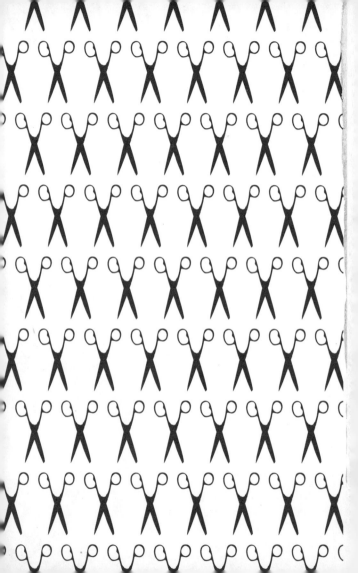

BEAUTY PARLOR WISDOM

By Risa Mickenberg
Photographs by Joanne Dugan
Design by Brian Lee Hughes

CHRONICLE BOOKS
SAN FRANCISCO

Copyright © 2006 by Risa Mickenberg.
Photographs copyright © 2006 by Joanne Dugan
Photography LLC.

Library of Congress Cataloging-in-Publication Data available.

ISBN: 0-8118-5211-3

Manufactured in China

Distributed in Canada by Raincoast Books
9050 Shaughnessy Street
Vancouver, British Columbia, V6P 6E5

10 9 8 7 6 5 4 3 2 1

Chronicle Books LLC
85 Second Street
San Francisco, California 94105

www.chroniclebooks.com

The quotes in this book were gleaned from conversations with stylists, barbers, manicurists, pedicurists, colorists, waxers, braiders, shampooers, mehndi artists, threaders, and fellow clients.

THANK YOU:

Al, Alicia, Alla, Alexander, Alexander, Andrea, Aneta, Angie, Ann, Beni, Blanca, Carol, Carrie, Cecilio, Celeste, Clarissa, David, Denise, Donna, Elena, Ella, Enis, Enrico, Faina, Flor, Franc, Frank, Georgia, Gilbert, Gina, Igor, James, Jeffrey, Jenee, Jeniette, Jennal, Ji, Jin, Jin Soon, Joe, John, Julie, Jyoti, Kanika, Kenneth, Kimberly, Kimiko, Kimmy, Lily, Lino, Lorraine, LuAnn, Luba, Luc, Margaret, Marta, Mathew, Max, Max, Maze, Mei Wei, Michael, Miguel, Mohammed, Naomi, Natasha, Olga, Paula, Pitti, Q, Rani, Raquel, RaRa, Ricky, Robert, Roxanne, Rumeka, Ruthie, Ruthy, Ryan, Saniye, Santy, Sexy Suga, Shibani, Starr, Tania, Tommy, Tyrone, Victor, Vishe, Wei Qing, Xiao Hui, Yoko, Zsuzsi

INTRODUCTION

Beauty is deep.

Not everyone goes to a therapist. But pretty much everyone, everywhere, at least gets a haircut.

It's no wonder that the connection we have with the Qs and Donnas and Pittis and Shibanis and Joes in our lives, the people who do our hair, our nails, our faces, our bodies, is so meaningful. These are intimate, ongoing, appointments wherein you command someone's complete and careful attention, in a soothing, cell phone–free world.

These are people who understand our cowlicks and our weird hair patches. They see our roots. They wrangle our toenails. They see us at our worst and make the best of us.

It goes far beyond maintenance. It's about the power of transformation. We go to them when we want to change. When we break up. When we get married. When we change jobs. When we're ill. When we want to become a new person. As we grow, as we age, as we reinvent ourselves, they make it happen for us. They are visionaries who see us not as we are, but as what we can pull off.

No wonder we are so very grateful to them. No wonder we hang on their every word.

They get our husbands back. They get us the gig, the job, the co-op, the girl. They're our accomplices in deception, in seduction, in reconciliation. We trust them with our most intimate secrets. They know when we're waxing for a tryst. They know what we're covering up. They see us without our faces on. Our confessors and our collaborators: they disguise, emphasize, dramatize. Draped in smocks, baptized in sinks, we dish the dirt. They hide our roots. They hold our hands.

These places are our modern sweat lodges, where we share the company of women, or men, in heated, close quarters. Our time there in chairs and on tables becomes a regular appointment for us to look in the mirror to decide whether we like what we see.

We leave with product in our hair and peace in our hearts. Feeling cleansed, made over. Like a new You.

Beauty has the power to change us, and, in turn, our lives. As one eyebrow threader said, "You change one thing, it changes everything."

And isn't that the meaning of life? To find beauty in ourselves, in the world, and in others? As one hairdresser put it: "Some people try to convince you they're ugly. It's your job not to let them."

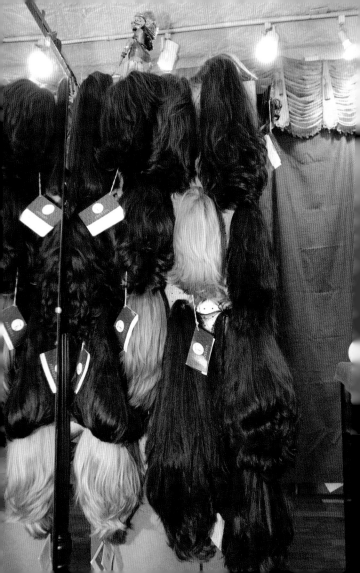

There are two schools of beauty—acceptance and denial.

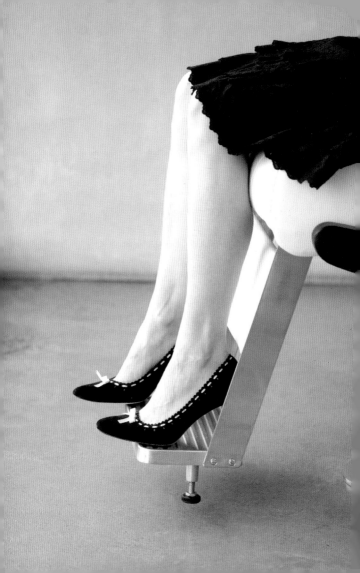

On universal weaknesses:

Everybody gets happy when someone beautiful is nice to them.

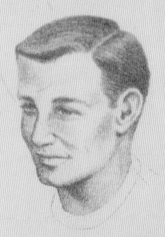

The Businessman's

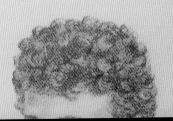

On lipstick and lovers:

If you
don't know
immediately,
it takes forever
to find the
right one.

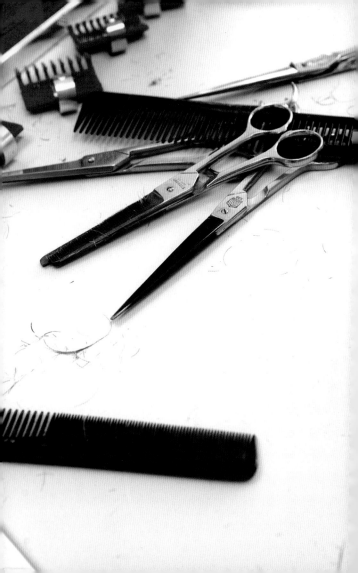

On diplomacy:

Never try to
come between
a woman
and her ideal
haircut.

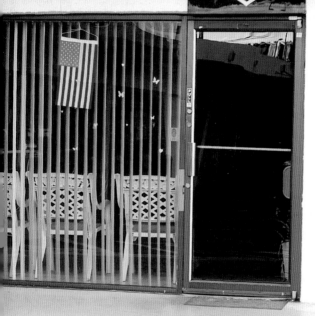

BeautySalon

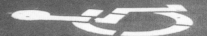

On rage:

Your boyfriend's driving always drives you crazy.

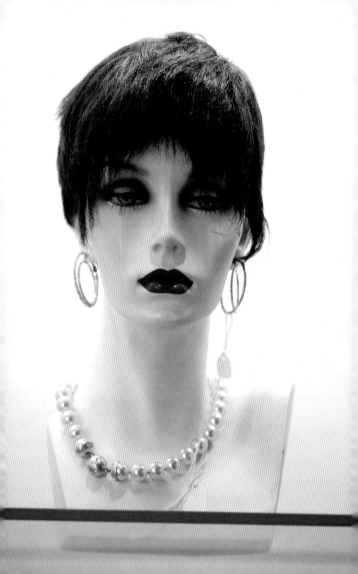

On Darwinism:

Sometimes being totally useless works for you.

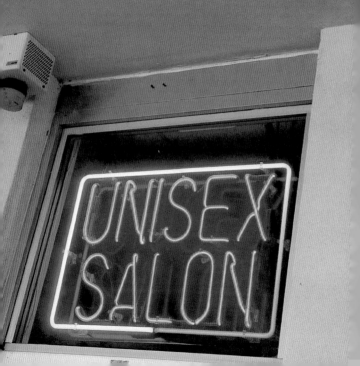

On being decisive:

If you don't have an opinion, you wind up with something you don't want.

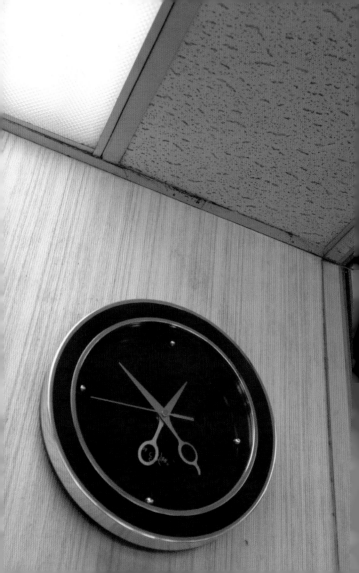

On family planning:

We were all accidents. Now they're all on purpose.

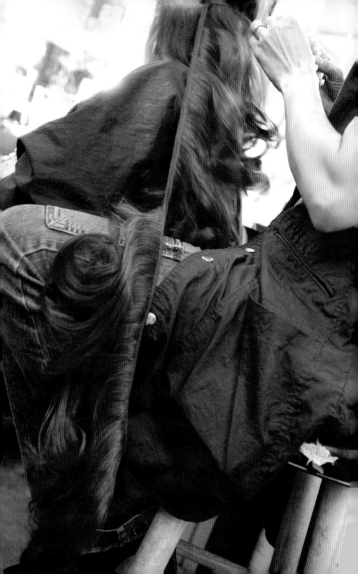

On goals:

Start at the ends and work your way back.

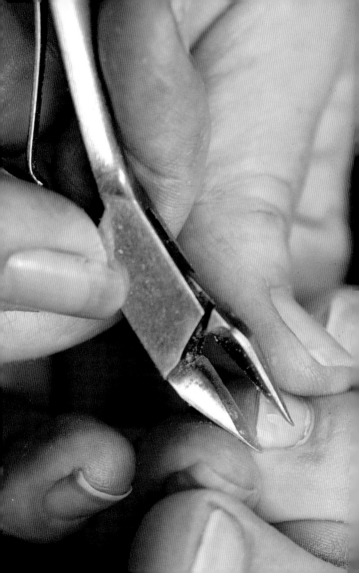

When times are bad, nails suffer.

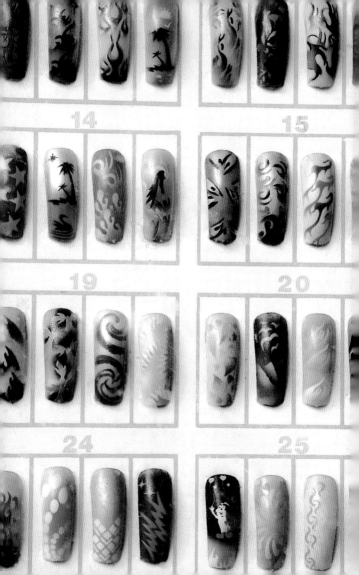

On making judgments:

The color of someone's skin doesn't tell you nearly as much about them as the color of their nail polish.

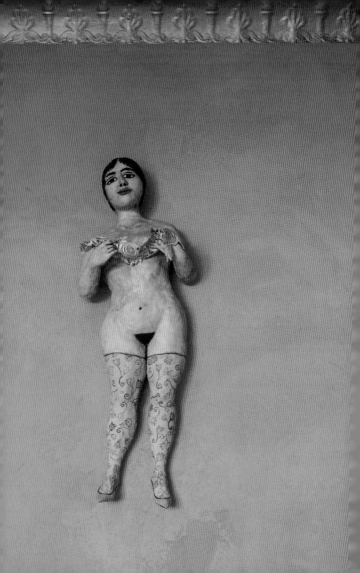

On relaxation:

Men go to strippers. Women get pedicures.

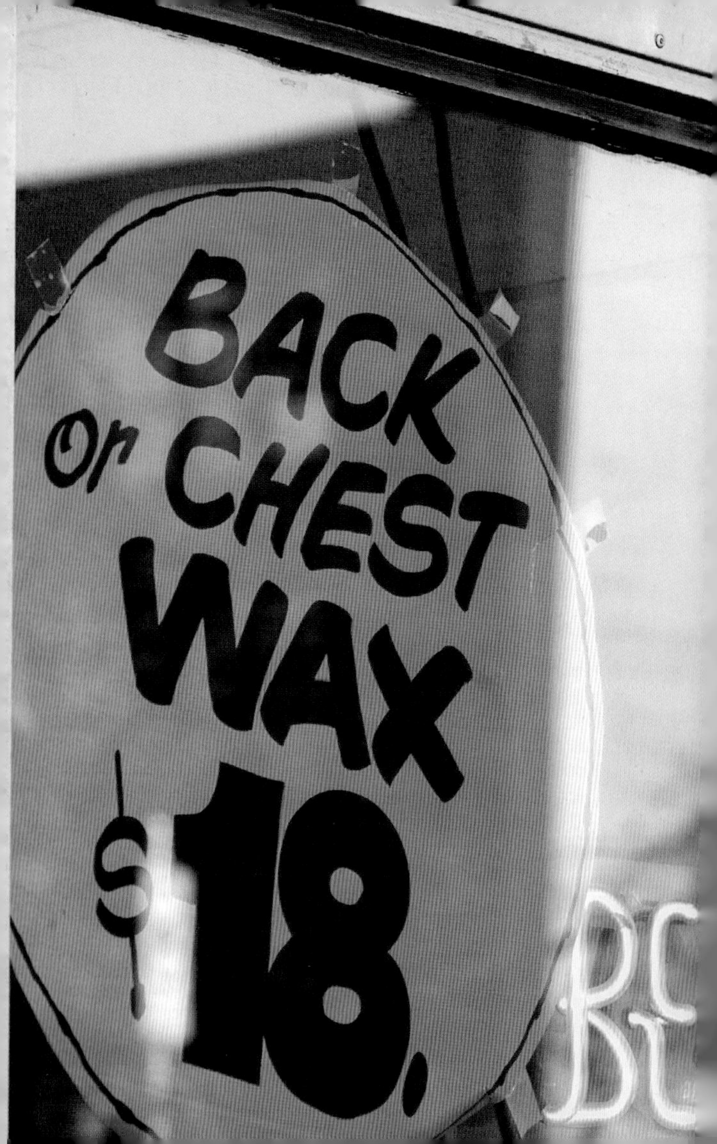
BACK
Or CHEST
WAX
$18.

People are more naturally one side or another.

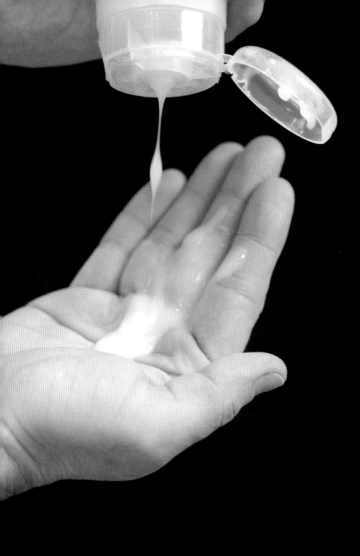

On men:

Women never fall asleep in the chair.

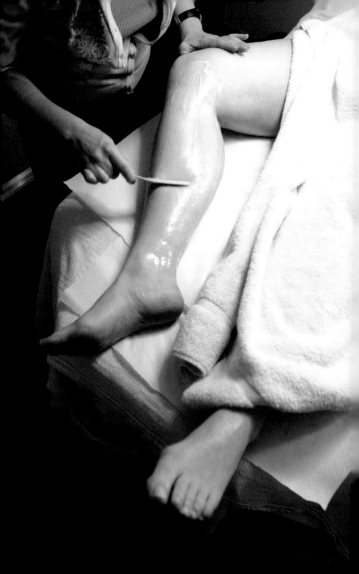

A man likes you to be cleaner than he is.

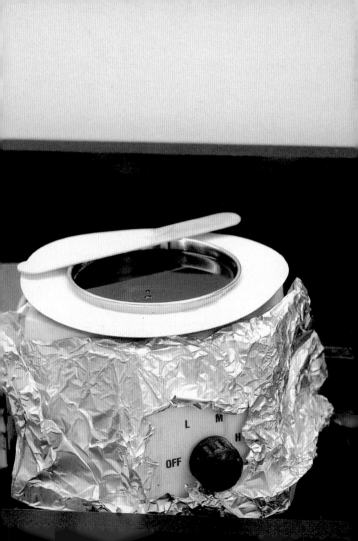

On L.A.:

Here,
it's pussy,
pussy,
pussy all day.

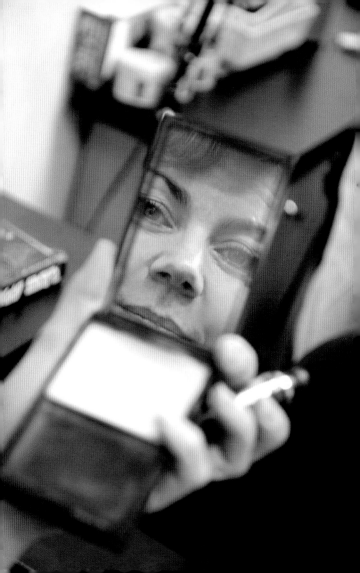

On true colors:

Women will lie to you about everything except your lipstick.

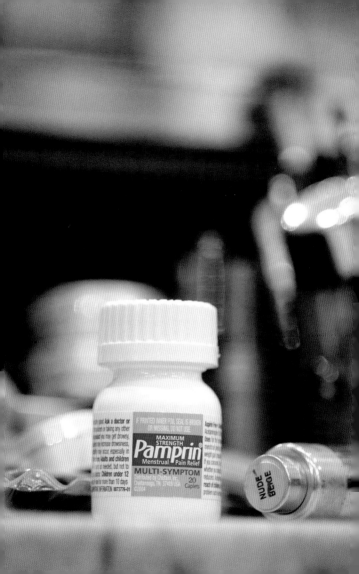

On size:

Big baby
is good,
but not in
a walk up.

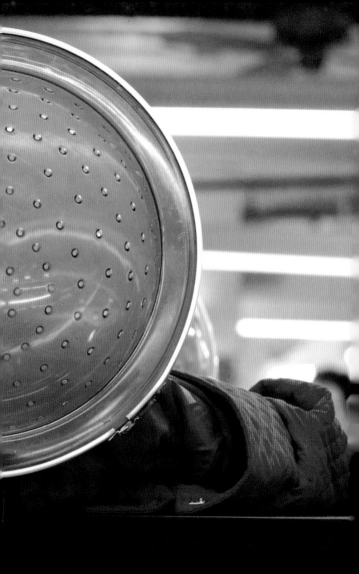

On relativity:

Never have
a handbag
bigger than
your ass.

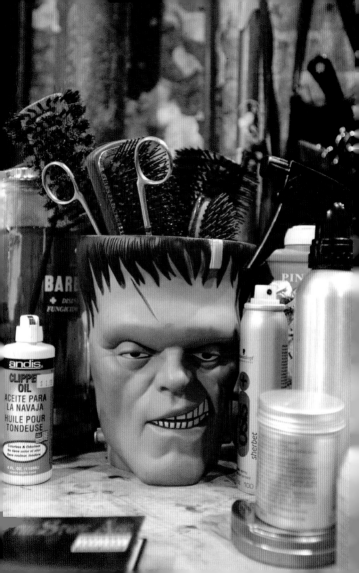

On salesmanship:

To sell someone something, they have to fall in love with you or be scared of you.

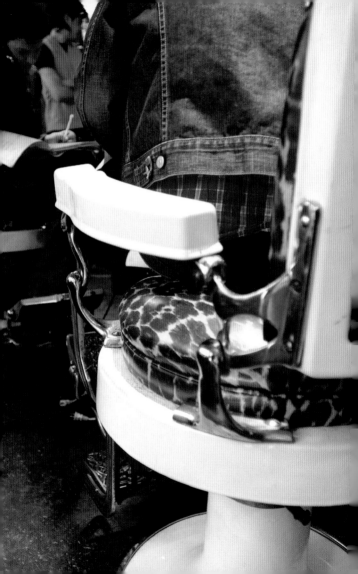

On behavior modification:

My friend is lesbian. She get no gifts. So she say no more lesbian.

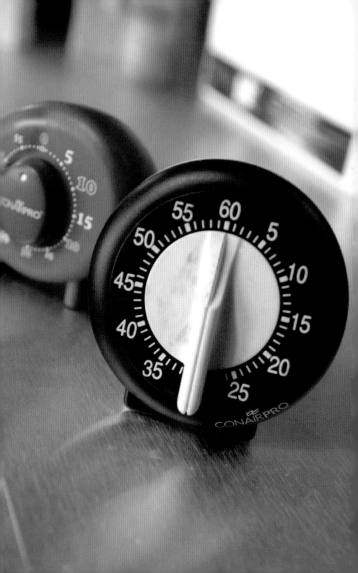

On patience:

The best way
to get a house
is to wait for
someone
to die.

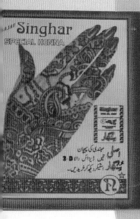

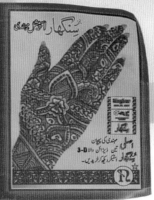

On proposals:

Listen to me—
Get yourself
pregnant.

$ 18

15

20 &UP

$ 10

15

$ 50

On paranoia:

You get money,
you get
suspicious.

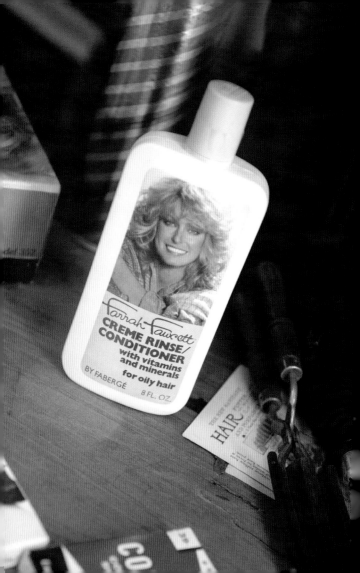

On communication:

People ask
for one thing
but what they
really want
is something
else.

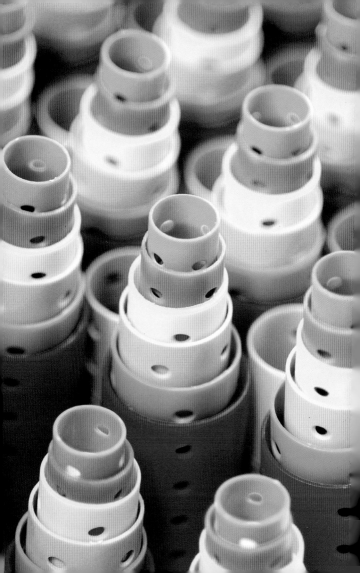

On depression:

Unhappy
people never
like their hair.

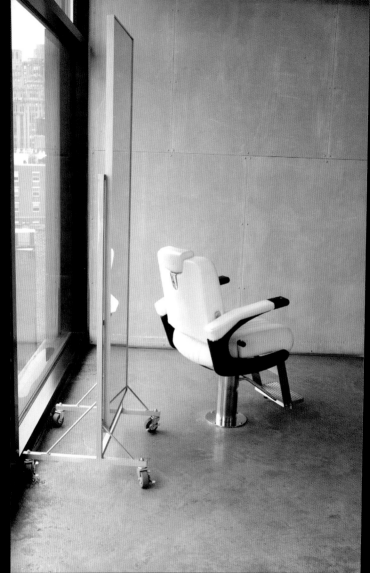

On Donald Trump:

One person,
lotta money.
Other person,
no money.
That's life.

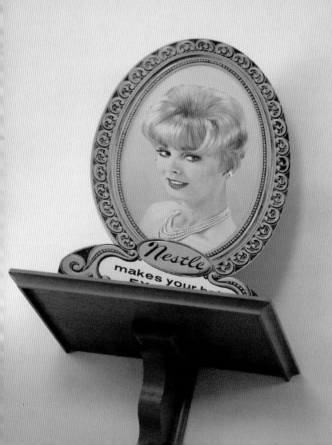

On standards:

You always want to look good enough to feel comfortable running into your ex.

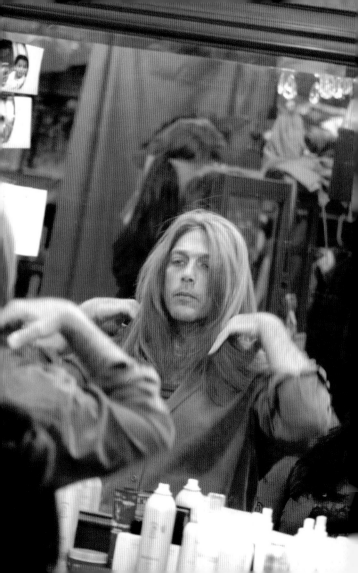

On the impermanence of permanents:

You can't change who you are.

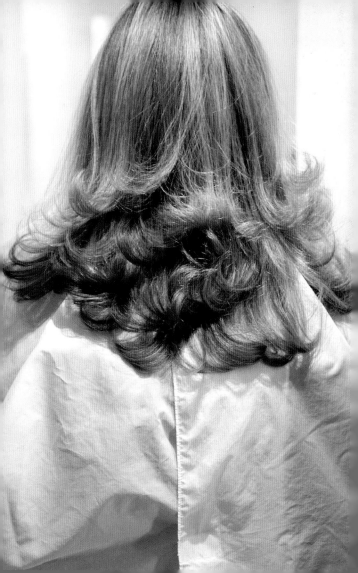

On three-ways:

One woman
always cries.

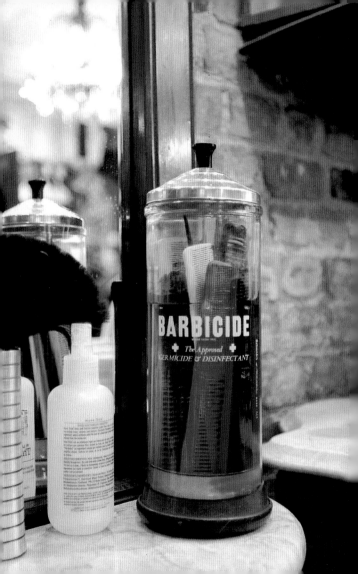

On the final stage of loss:

My hair used
to be a vestige
of what it used
to be.
Now it just is
what it is.

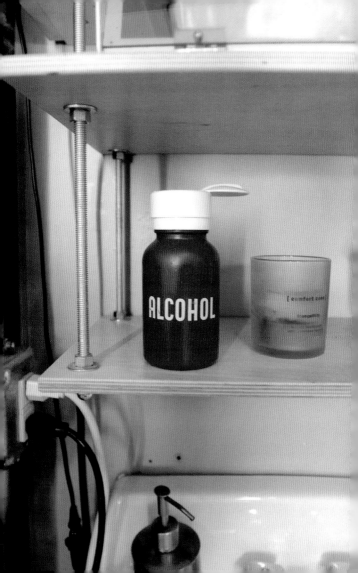

On holding your tongue:

If someone's getting stupid, don't get smart.

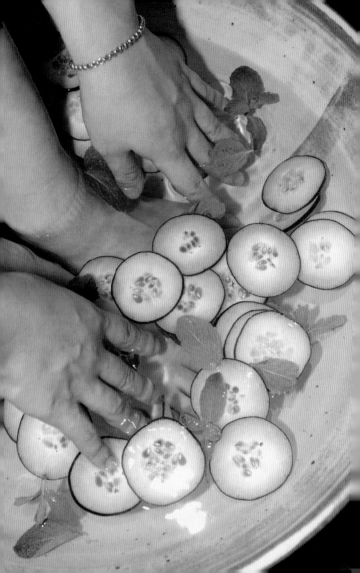

On manicure parties:

When I was
little girl,
nails were
for scratching
your sister.

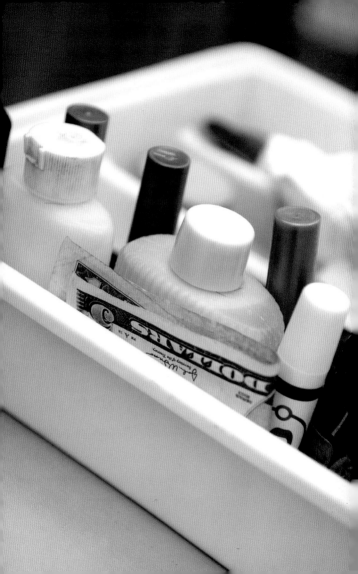

On power:

You can
control people
with very small
amounts of
money.

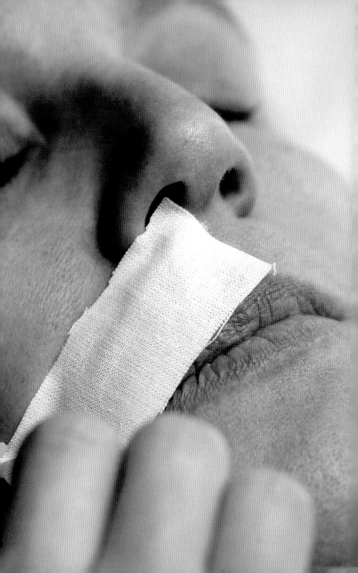

On virility:

Good news is...
woman with
moustache
have bigger
orgasm.

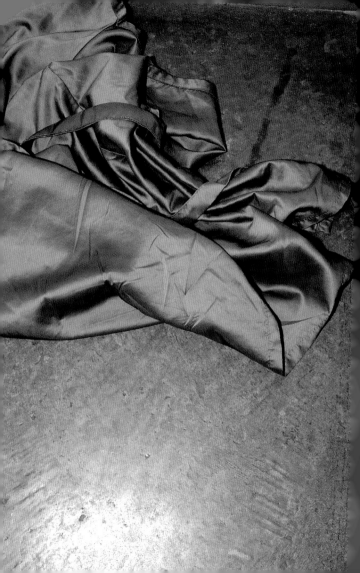

On intellectualizing:

We decide
with our heart.
Then we use
our brain to
clean up the
mess.

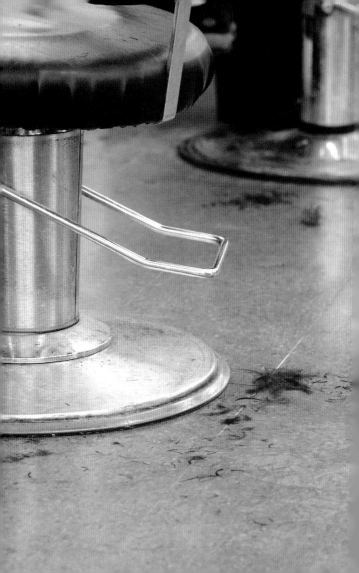

On comb-overs:

You don't put
them down to
make them
change.
You say bald
is sexy.

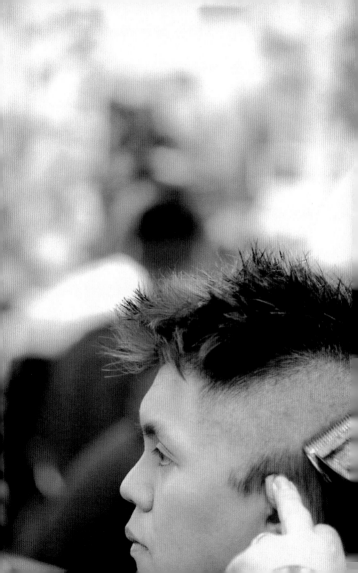

On Lite FM:

You play crazy music you get crazy people.

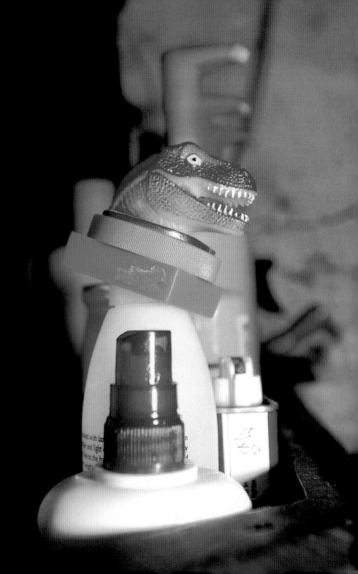

On loving your work:

You don't work
with the hair.
You play with
the hair.

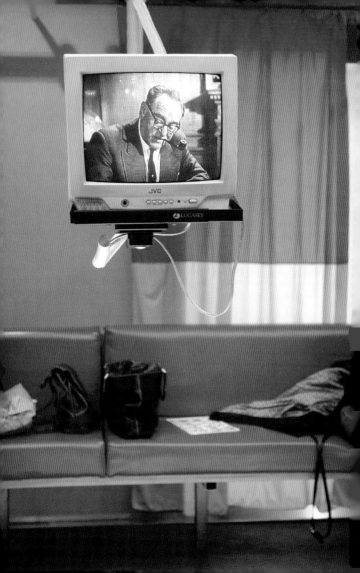

On control:

Women,
they talk.
Men,
they listen.

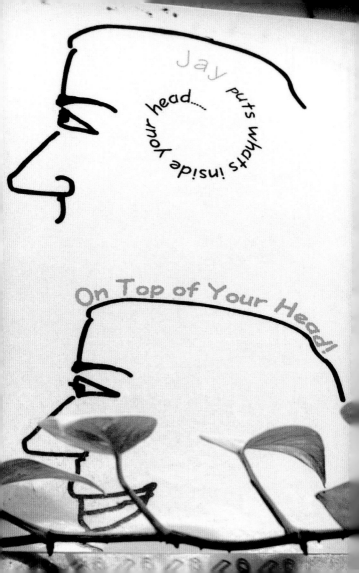

On interpretation:

People think
everything
will translate.
They're wrong.

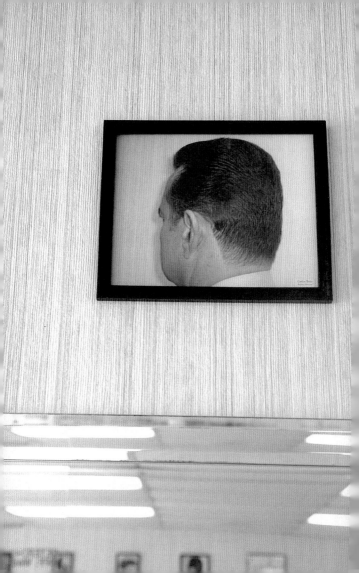

On flirting:

Men need to feel jealous every once in a while.

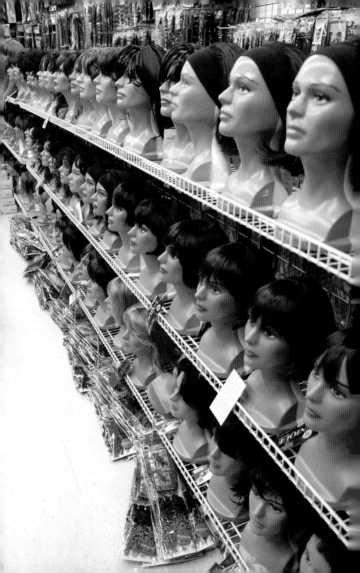

On clairvoyance:

You can see
a person's
whole life
in their hair.

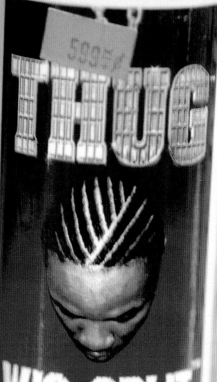

On scruffiness:

Some people can't pull it off.

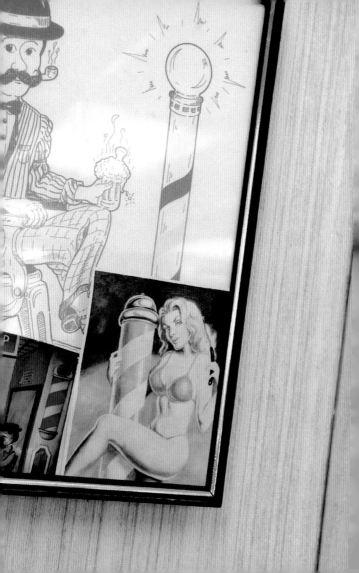

On professionalism:

They're not supposed to massage your boobs.

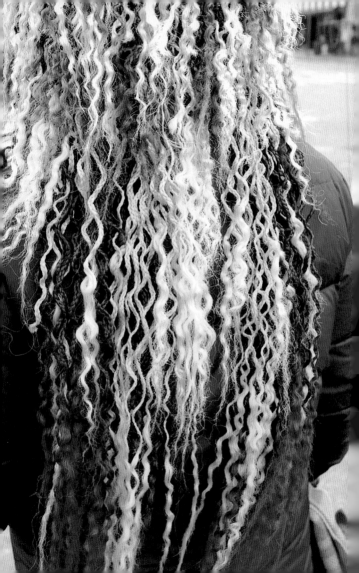

Men are easy.
Women are
complicated.
Bald men
are most
complicated.

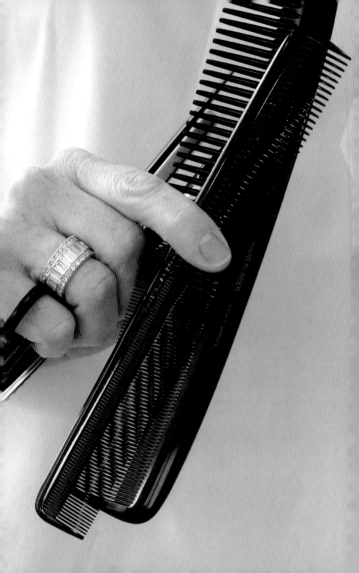

On divorce settlements:

Keep it.
You can always
give it back.

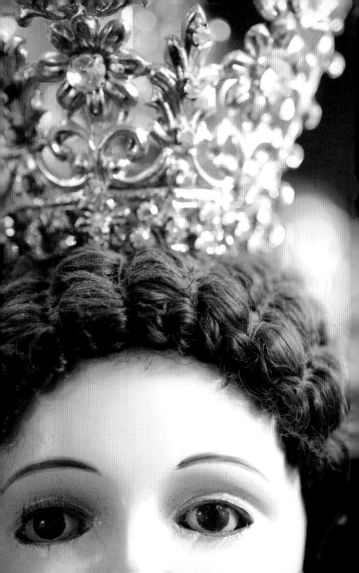

On faith:

Some people
try to convince
you they're
ugly.
It's your
job not to
let them.

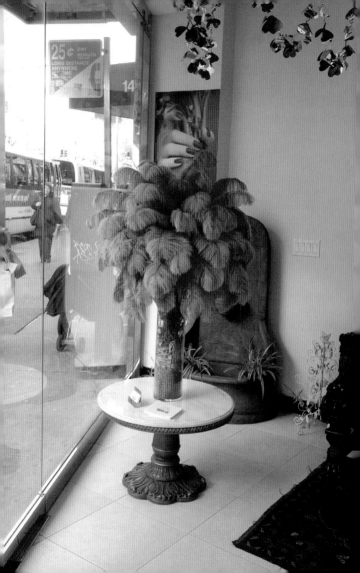

On floral arrangements:

Please.
No more kale
in bouquets.

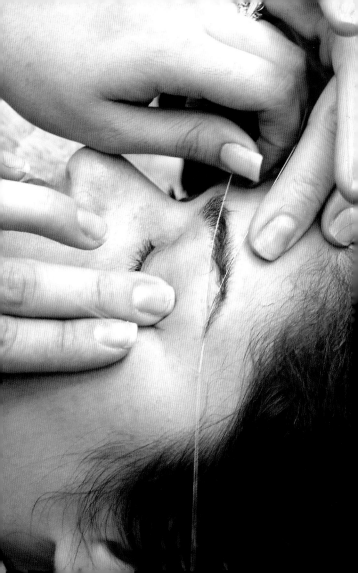

On effort:

You change
one thing,
it changes
everything.

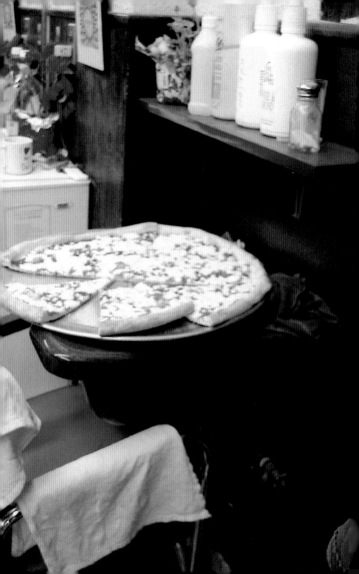

On preventing hangovers:

A couple hours before you drink, eat some prickly pear.

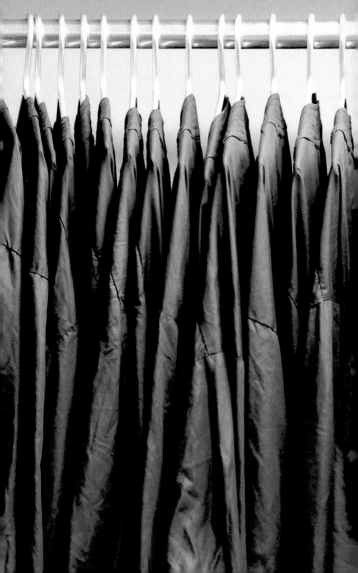

On ruts:

With some
people it's
always like
last time.

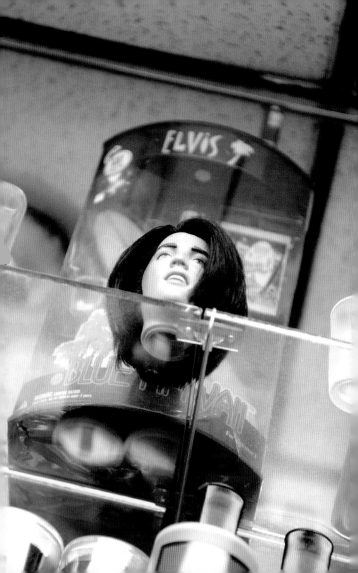

On militarization:

When they cut Elvis' hair, it changed the world.

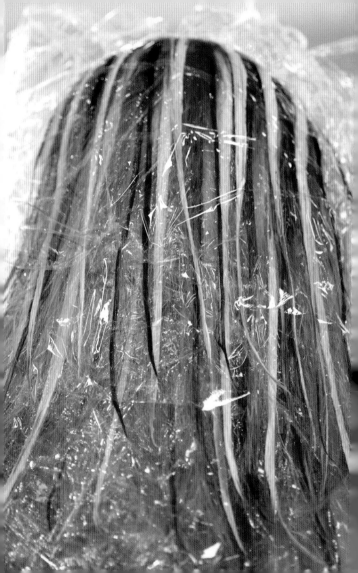

On quantum theory:

Your hair is
a microcosm
of your head.

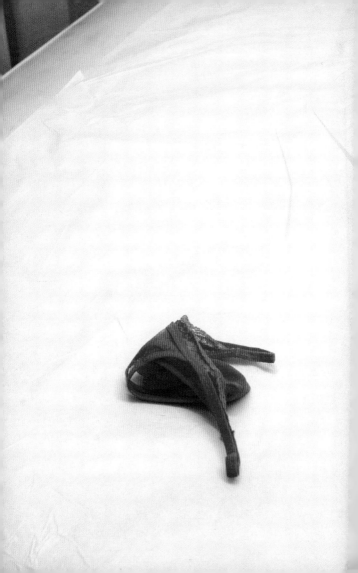

On porno films:

Hi-def video
is great for
business.

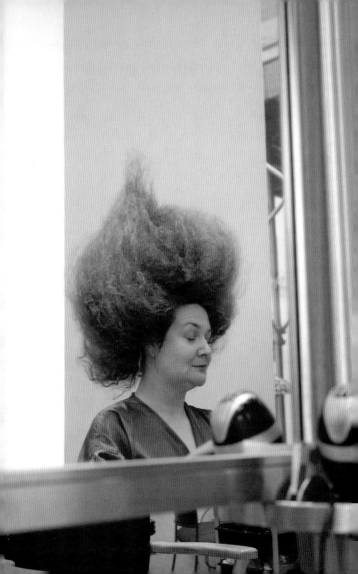

On courage:

I love people
who get crazy
haircuts.

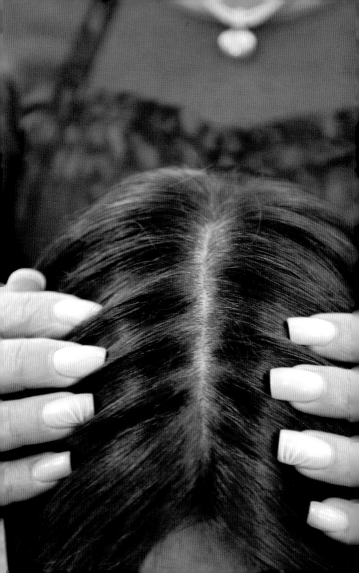

On the curiousness of criticism:

You never
know who's
going to get
picky.

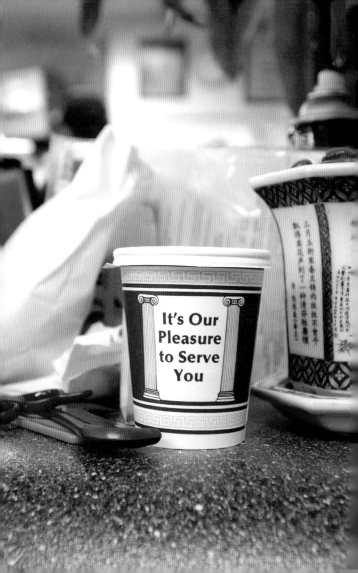

A serious tip:

Put pee pee
on the face.

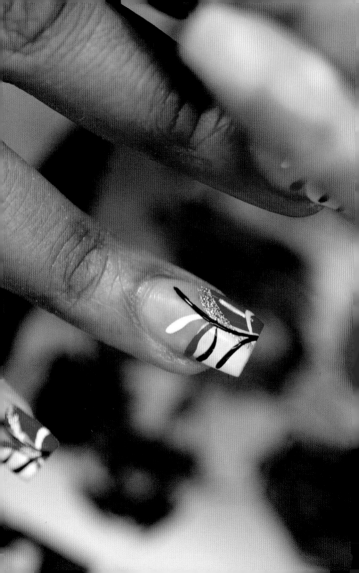

Women like
the very long
nails. Men
don't care.

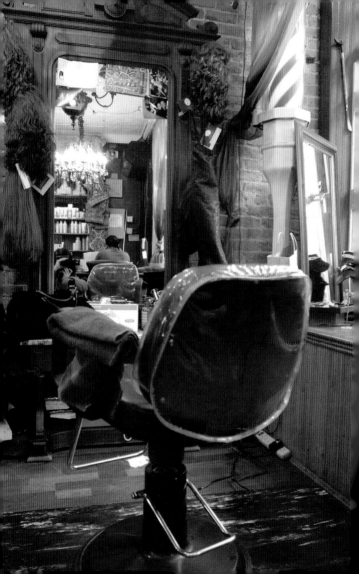

Final cut:

The last thing they do after you die, is your hair.

Concentrate equilibrant

Ingredients: Limnanthus Alba (Mea)
• Cyclomethicone • Ricinu Con
Chinensis (Jojoba) Seed Oil • Me
Piperita (Peppermint) Oil • Tocce
• Guaiacol • Bisabolol • Ascor
Ascorbate • Tocopherol • Isobuty
• Phenoxyethanol • Isopropylen

CAUTION: For external use only. A
wounds or broken skin./PRECAUT
externe. Ne pas appliquer sur les
cutanées./PRECAUCIÓN: Para us
ojos, membranas mucosas, herida
Anwendung: Nicht in die Augen ur
oder wunden Hautstellen fernhalt
usare su occhi, membrane mucos

Aveda Corporation, Dixe, Minnesota
London W1K 3BO Made in US 66 96
www.aveda.com   A5FC/A5FC/SVL/

BEAUTIFYING

On nature:

There's no
harmony in
plastic
surgery.

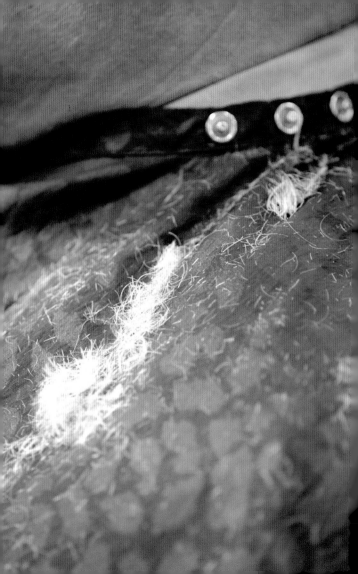

On snobbery:

Old money
was once
new money.

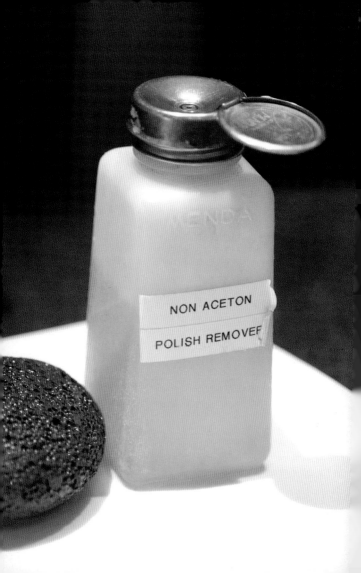

On aging:

World-weary is
a valid look.

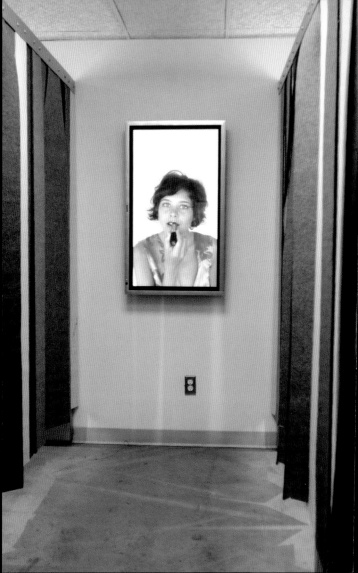

On keeping the peace:

No talk.
Watch TV.

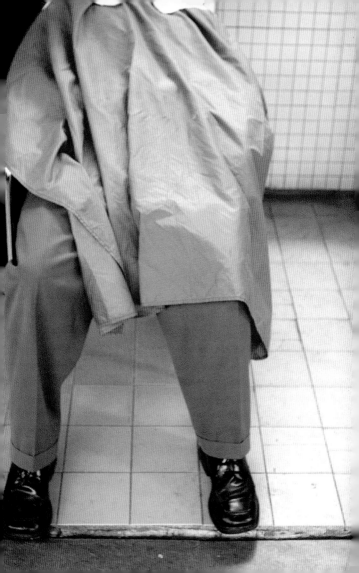

On contrast:

The darker
you go, the
lighter
the light is.

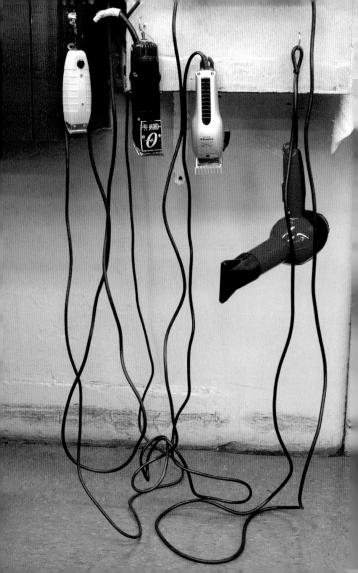

On job security:

There's always gonna be hair.

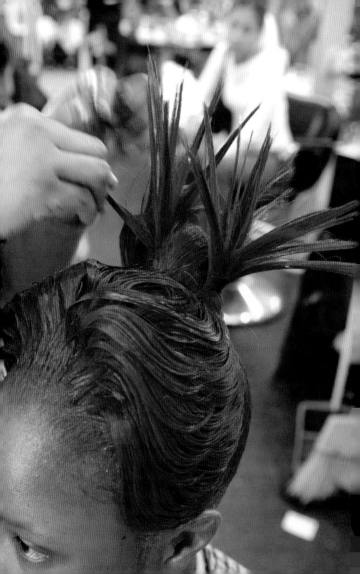

On changing identity:

Curly hair can just become all of a sudden straight.

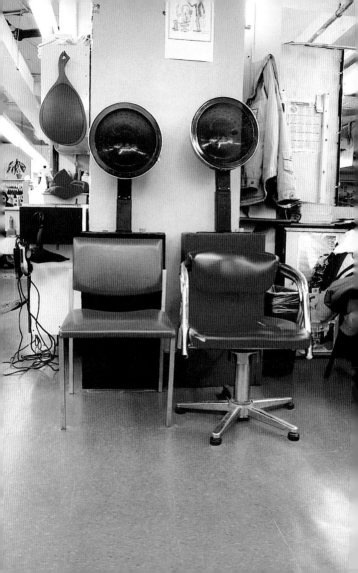

On accessorizing:

The eyebrows usually match the pubic hair.

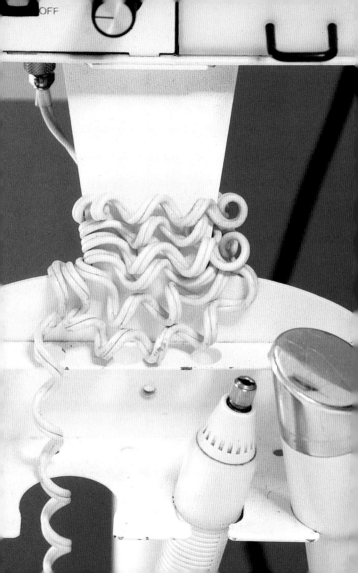

Every woman has one crazy hair growing out of her face.

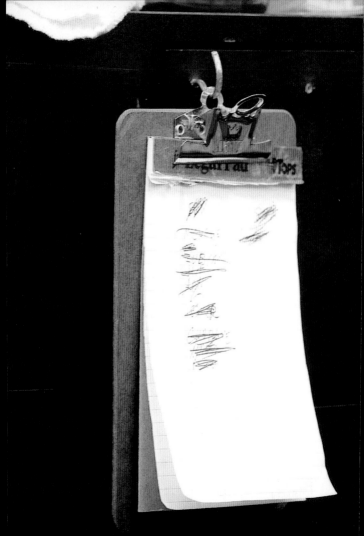

The equation:

If you don't care about money, you don't get money.

HAIRPIECES
by Appointment Only

before

after

ask for Mr Albert

On hypochondria:

It's okay
to dream.

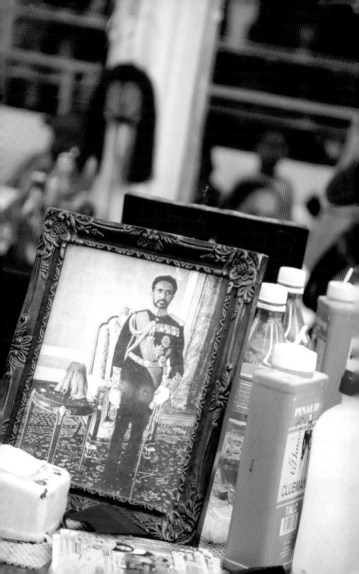

On stroking:

I'm not about
the truth.
I'm about
making you
feel good
about yourself.

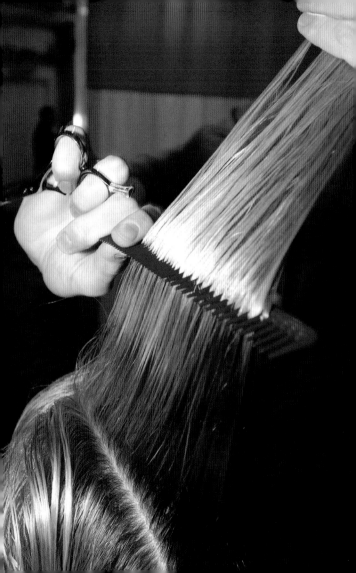

On fatalism:

Bad hair never
looks good
and good hair
never looks
bad.

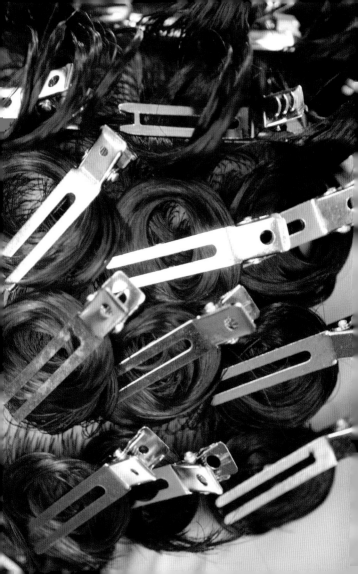

On commitment:

Don't start or you'll never be able to stop.

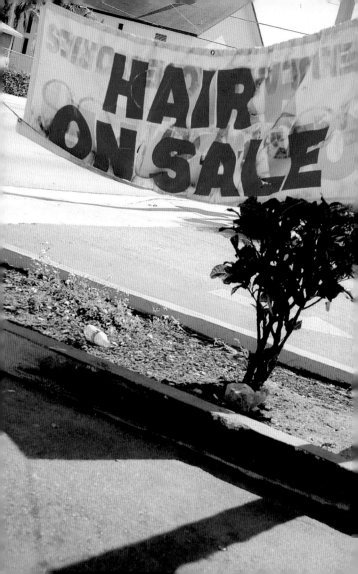

On perceived differences:

You say
natural.
I say lazy.

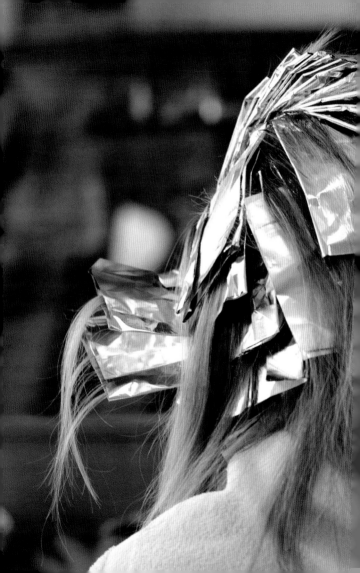

On timing:

You go before you're set, you ruin everything.

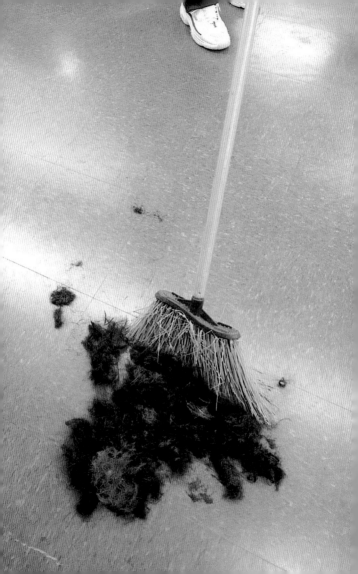

On grudges:

You never
forget your
first hate,
either.

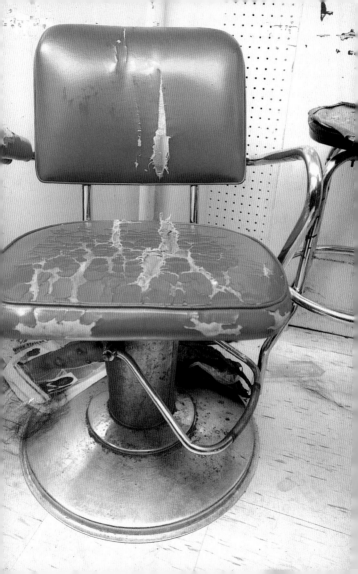

On ugly days:

Looking bad doesn't make you invisible. You just look bad.

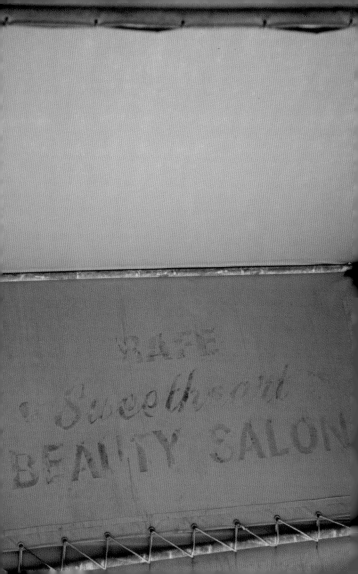

On recreational use:

We had so many friends when we all did drugs.

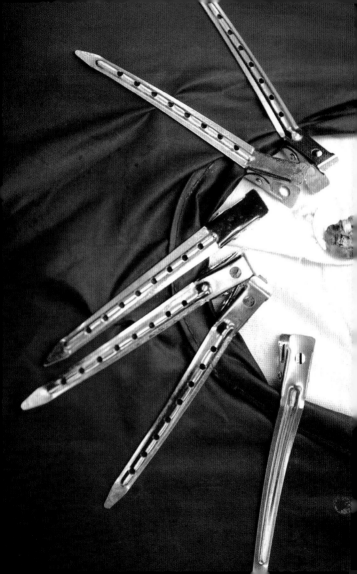

A warning:

You never
want to get
on the wrong
side of a tiny
Japanese
gay man.

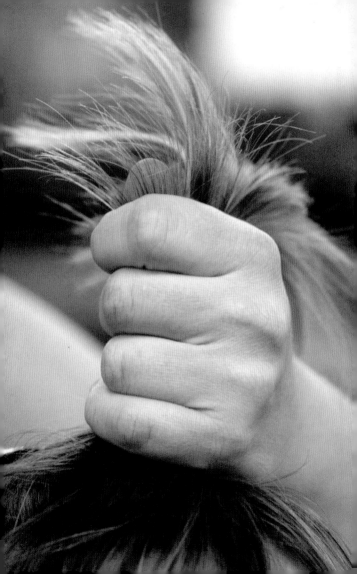

On tenacity:

Maybe you
not as strong
as you hair.

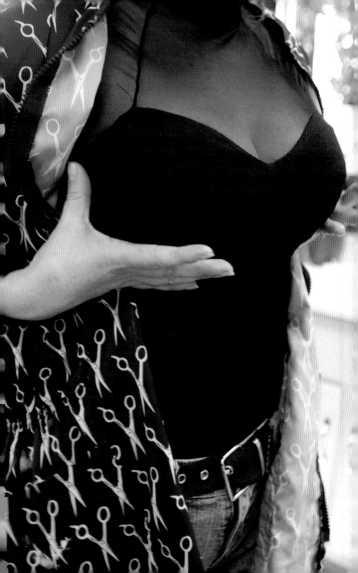

On attraction:

Sexy is highly subjective.

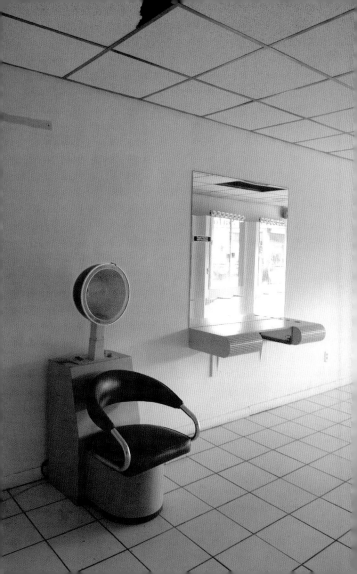

On surrendering:

You don't lose your looks. You give them up.

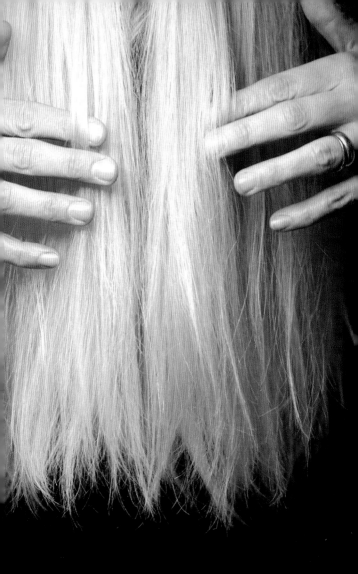

On growth:

It's all about growing out well.

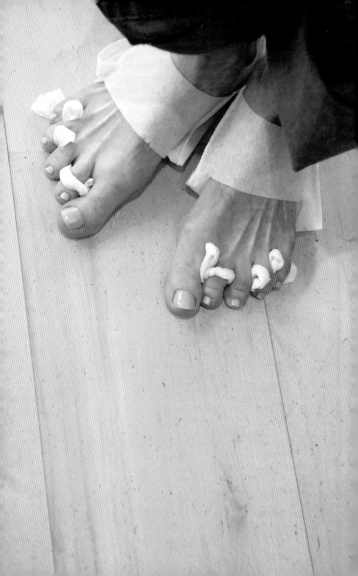

Be careful you nails.

YOU'RE GORGEOUS

Sarah Malarkey, Felix Andrew, DeMane Davis,
The Mickenbergs, Libby Brockhoff, Ludovic and Hugo
Moulin, The Dugan Family, Cisca Gia, The Hughes Family,
Cat Schwartz, Christine Earle, Matt Robinson, Miami Ad
School, Tim Stacheki at Nikon Professional Services

and

Adams West, Artisan Spa, Astor Place Hairstylist Inc.,
Mei Yue Chen Hair Removal, Creative Concept Beauty
Studio, Sip N Snip, Adams West Unisex, Little Tony's Elvis,
Unisex Hair, Beauty and Youth Spa, Carousel Salon,
Platinum Styles, Little Haiti Flea Market, Cutting Room,
Joe's Foodland, Santy Hair Salon, Freddie Lucero Salon,
Red Rose Beauty Salon, Jeniette New York, Jeffrey Indyke
Hair Salon, Donna McNally Salon, Carsten Hair Salon, Jin
Soon Natural Hand and Foot Spa, Eva Of New York, Rose
Hair Braiding, John Barrett Salon at Bergdorf Goodman,
Mud Honey Salon, Bumble and Bumble Downtown Salon,
Charles Worthington LLC, Circle Beauty, Golden Coiffures
Salon, Barber Shop and Stylist, Joe's Beauty Supply, Oscar
Bond Salon, Q Hair, Think Pink, Nice Nails, Fine Nails,
Sparkle Beauty Studio, many others and all aesthetes
everywhere.

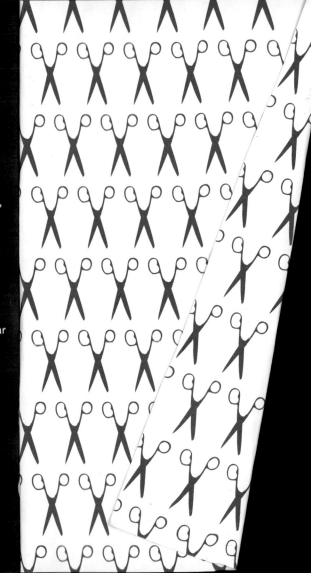

As you leave:

Be careful
you nails.

YOU'RE GORGEOUS

Sarah Malarkey, Felix Andrew, DeMane Davis,
The Mickenbergs, Libby Brockhoff, Ludovic and Hugo
Moulin, The Dugan Family, Cisca Gia, The Hughes Family,
Cat Schwartz, Christine Earle, Matt Robinson, Miami Ad
School, Tim Stacheki at Nikon Professional Services

and

Adams West, Artisan Spa, Astor Place Hairstylist Inc.,
Mei Yue Chen Hair Removal, Creative Concept Beauty
Studio, Sip N Snip, Adams West Unisex, Little Tony's Elvis,
Unisex Hair, Beauty and Youth Spa, Carousel Salon,
Platinum Styles, Little Haiti Flea Market, Cutting Room,
Joe's Foodland, Santy Hair Salon, Freddie Lucero Salon,
Red Rose Beauty Salon, Jeniette New York, Jeffrey Indyke
Hair Salon, Donna McNally Salon, Carsten Hair Salon, Jin
Soon Natural Hand and Foot Spa, Eva Of New York, Rose
Hair Braiding, John Barrett Salon at Bergdorf Goodman,
Mud Honey Salon, Bumble and Bumble Downtown Salon,
Charles Worthington LLC, Circle Beauty, Golden Coiffures
Salon, Barber Shop and Stylist, Joe's Beauty Supply, Oscar
Bond Salon, Q Hair, Think Pink, Nice Nails, Fine Nails,
Sparkle Beauty Studio, many others and all aesthetes
everywhere.

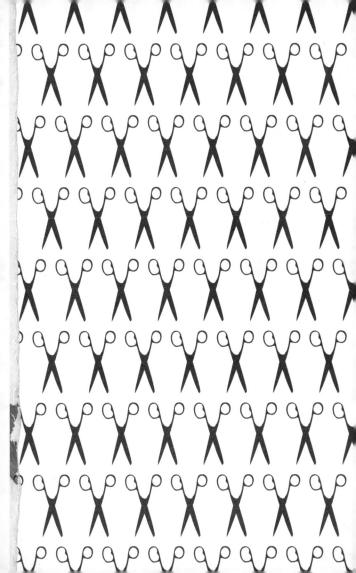

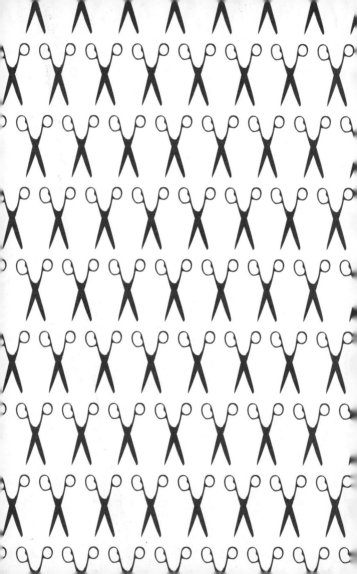